Reclaiming My Time

A Practical Guide to Self-Care

Jeanette Ferrell

Published by FastPencil Publishing

First Edition

http://fp.fastpencil.com

Printed in the United States of America

Table of Contents

The universe has a way of pulling your coat tail to get your attention. Well for me, it pushed me down, face first in the mud. Seeds grow towards the sunlight. Those sprouts push through and struggle through the darkness and dirt towards the light to become what they were meant to be. For this, I thank the UnIverse! To my partner in love and life, my wife, T.J. I thank you for your reverence, patience, love, support, but most of all I thank the Most High for your existence. To the people that make up my tribe, thank you for sitting through those grueling conversations about all the creative messes I find myself in. To my sisters in life, Tasha and Tasharia, I thank you for walking this journey with me no matter the starting points, the detours and traffic we've sat in, your contribution is appreciated. To my parents, I love you! Shout out to both of you for creating a legend!

This book is dedicated to the work and love of life of my OG, Margaret Jean Irvin! I love you Granny! This book is also written and dedicated to the women that are at revolutionary points in their lives! Change becomes you!

Introduction

If you ask the average person their thoughts about self-care, many will say it's something that they haven't even thought about. What's even more surprising is that our society teaches us that self- care is selfish, overly indulgent and arrogant. This belief intensifies when it comes to women taking out time for themselves. Women are expected to be the nurtures, problem solvers, mothers, wives and God in human form to everyone and everything but themselves. How dare we steal a moment for ourselves after living and working under mundane conditions, lower pay wages, and heightened distress all while staring down the barrel of potential perils of violent conditions, harassment, disobedient/difficult children, and an inattentive/unappreciative spouse.

As a woman standing at the crossroads of intersectionality of being an African-American woman, who's a single mother that happens to identify as lesbian and as more spiritual than religious, I can recall several occurrences of my life that have threatened my personal dignity, character and minimized my confidence. Change came when I realized that all of these things depleted me emotionally, physically, mentally, and sometimes financially. I accepted that the time had come in my life to seek balance and put myself first.

If you've ever flown on a plane, just as you're all snuggled in your seat with your belt fastened; the flight attendant prepares the cabin for take-off and begin to provide instructions on how to survive should optimal flying conditions change. Of those instructions the most important thing she says isn't how to activate your flotation device. It's, "...should there be a change in cabin pressure an oxygen mask will deploy, place the mask securely on yourself before assisting other passengers." Who knew that the most critical component in a secure and vividly lived life, would come from a flight attendant? Once you begin to put yourself first, and care for yourself properly, it's as if the universe opens up and showers your life with reflections of that love and care. Here love and care are used synonymously. Here you will find practical notions, considerations, and to-do's that guide you...women standing at blurring 'intersectionalities'....to self-care.

Chapter 1: You Better Find Your Ass: Self Preservation

In A *Burst of Light: Essays*, Audre Lorde proclaimed, *"Caring for myself isn't self-indulgence, it is self-preservation, and that is an act of political warfare."* For women of color, particularly black women, this rings true. According to, *feministwire.com*, "Statistics *about black women's health are dismal. In regards to our mental health, our depression rate is estimated to be 50% higher than white women's.* Within the realm of physical health, *black women face particular challenges around diabetes, heart disease, and high blood pressure. One in 4 black women over the age of 55 have diabetes.[i] [http://www.thefeministwire.com/2012/11/subversive-self-care-centering-black-womens-wellness/#_edn1]* Black women die *from heart disease more than any other group in America.[ii] [http://www.thefeministwire.com/2012/11/ subversive-self-care-centering-black-womens-wellness/#_edn2] Health studies have shown that risk factors, which include a lack of exercise, poor eating habits, and high levels of stress, contribute to the development of these diseases. What's more, however, is that the stressful challenges that black women face as primary caregivers – mothers and other-mothers – and academics make this a serious issue that we need to unpack (Covington-Ward 2013). In light of these statistics, we have to recognize what's at stake in unpacking the wellness, life balance, and self-care needs of black women." Furthermore, in the article,* **Subversive Self-Care, Centering Black Women's Wellness**, *on feministwire.com, the expectations of the family can too heavily affect the health of women Dr. Tamara Beauboeuf-Lafontant, examines the strong black woman and describes the strong black woman as superwoman that is expected to endure extensive emotional, mental, and physical setbacks and difficulties and live a life of quality. (Beauboeuf-Lafonant, 2009: 2).*

Dr. Lafontant's claim asserts Ms. Lourdes proclamation and provides us the purpose for this societal practice...to discount and obscure Black women's experiences of suffering, acts of desperation and anger. Self-care has been many things for me. Early in my life self-care meant splurging and buying things I didn't necessarily need because I deserved it. As I grew a bit older self-care meant doing things for myself that I didn't normally do, like go to a new club or hang out with a new set of people. When 30 approached and I so desperately held on to my vanishing 20's, self-care had become something that "old people" did to slow down their aging process. To better care for myself meant acknowledging that I was getting old and certainly, what girl holding steadfast to her girlish charm would be willing to accept this horrid truth. It was then I stopped carving out time to care for myself, no matter how I defined it. Fast forward to the mid thirty's, add on elements of adulting, failed relationships, and job mediocrity; after making deposits in everything and everyone else, I found myself with insufficient amounts in my own 'mental' bank account. It was at this time that Ms. Lourdes's proclamation found its way in my head and changed my thinking. I had considered self-care many things, but never in my wildest thoughts would I have considered it an act of political warfare, an act of rebellion. How could getting mani/pedi's, massages, taking long candle filled soaks, and eating good food be revolutionary? Self-care was a survival method, an avoidance to aging, not a revolutionary act. I once relished in being on the receiving end of provided services instead of being the provider of those services. I, like many other women was caring for myself in spite of life and the intersectional –isms that left me in emotional and mental debt. I quickly found that caring for myself was leading me to financial woes that I simply couldn't afford. Suddenly, I couldn't afford to take care of myself in the ways I had grown accustomed. This sent me in a downward spiral to places that were lonely, dark and cold. I couldn't return there. I had to do something. I had to find a better way to care for myself. I had attached self-care to materialistic things. I had to improve my method of self-care so I detached MY self-care from capitalism. I had to be rich in spirit, mind, and health. I had to simply stop pouring into those institutions and people that not only refused to reciprocate the deposits, but refused to acknowledge the idea that it was imperative to my health and success as a productive member of society. I had to self-preserve without going bankrupt, so I abandoned my self-care as defined by the latest magazines and talk shows. I had arrived at the realization that I needed to recharge from the inequitable norms that slowly drilled away pieces of who I was...and was to become and that even the recharge itself was unequitable. I was in need of accessible self-care no matter how much money was in my wallet. In seeking equity outside of myself, I realized that I had to create equity within myself. It all started with me and the way I loved and cared for myself. Let's examine self-love to define "proper self-care". I believe self-care begins with self-love. It is impossible to properly care for yourself if you don't have a deep rooted love for yourself. When discussing self-love, I'm talking beyond the surface. Sure, going to the doctor for preventative care, exercising and eating right so that you live a long good life shows that you love yourself, but I want to dig a bit deeper. Self-love can be defined as doing, speaking and living in a matter that ensures your health, sanity, progress, and productivity. This includes investing in yourself, learning and studying yourself, setting boundaries, forgiving yourself, saying the hard things, walking toward those things that scare you, and removing yourself from situations and people that don't serve you. Loving yourself helps you avoid situations and people that prevent you from caring properly for yourself. Thus, proper self-care can then be defined as the thoughts and actions that reinforces health, self-worth, self-esteem, and confidence. Society tell us (women) that we should give willingly and freely of ourselves to everyone but ourselves. Women are expected to stretch themselves thin to serve populations that find it difficult to acknowledge them, to honor them and apply equity to their lives. If we are giving of ourselves in this manner then how do we survive? How do we establish and maintain a high quality of life? The answer is simple... Self-Preservation. It is fine time for women to do things that aid in their preservation of self. Now I know you may be asking, "How do I preserve myself with 3 children, a full time job, school, and the part time job I just picked up on the weekends because Little Susan is now in gymnastics on Mondays, Wednesdays and Fridays?" While there is no cliff's notes or microwaveable way to self-preservation there are steps you can take. The first step in self-preservation is understanding that it's crucial to your existence that you care for yourself physically and psychically. Decompressing is useful in reflecting over your day, your actions and your words. Create a space that is isolated safe, quiet and healing. This space can be in anywhere in your home or outside in your yard. This space is yours, where you alone should retreat to have those moments to yourself to assess your daily productivity and mistakes. Focus on what you actually had control over and what was beyond that control. Plan to improve your day by amending those things that you had control over that you would do better or differently. It's important to be aware that not all things will work according to plan or in our time, and there is absolutely nothing you can do about that, so take care not to beat yourself up about it.

After you've created a space to decompress, carve out time to enjoy your space and learn more about you and what makes you tick. Often time, we think we really know ourselves. We know our favorite colors, foods, even the guilty pleasures and secrets we harbor. But how many of us are taking the time to get to know ourselves as we age, as we recover from grief and heart ache? My guess is not too many of us really know who we are because we don't have or make time to get reacquainted. Give yourself 10-30 minutes per day to just sit, journal or think. This is the time to talk to yourself without people perceiving you as weird or "crazy". It is also a good time to have a good cry and deeply examine the feelings you have and why. If you find that you can't give yourself 10-30 minutes in one setting take 5 minutes, and add a minute to those blocks each day until you have achieved a full 30 minutes per day.

The next step in self-preservation is to take time for you EACH DAY without feeling guilty. YOU Deserve This! I understand that if YOU don't pick up and drop off the cupcakes for your daughter for gymnastics class by 5:30, the instructor and other parents will deem you a bad or lazy parent, and well you just can't have that right? Wrong! Let them think what they will. The world won't end if the cupcakes arrive at 6pm instead. Self-Preservation is the first law of nature. It ensures that you survive. Certainly there should be no guilt in surviving.

The final step in self-preservation boldly saying, "NO" and meaning it. No, is a complete sentence. It doesn't require an explanation. The law of self-preservation says that people have the right to guard the sanctity and value of their life through any means necessary. Sometimes "NO" is that means. Many women feel pressure when saying "no", and this is symbolic of the lack of freedom in given relationships. We as women, feel pressure for NOT making sacrifices for others. Saying "no" to things that you don't want to do or don't have time to do provides internal freedom. Be aware that burdening ourselves with the problems of others is easy to do. For women of all cultures, it's expected. Helping others is embedded and reinforced in our cultural upbringing, however, there are limits. Freedom is obtained by setting boundaries. Once you've spent some time with yourself, you will find that you've learned several things. Of those things, new boundaries will begin to form and anyone that cross that boundary will need to be informed of the consequences of crossing that boundary in the future. It feels good to establish a boundary and you yourself operate within that boundary. This gives you the power to enforce those boundaries. Failing to declare and enforce those boundaries leaves us open to what I like to call, the Succubus Ones, a more common reference however, is energy vampires. People, rather intentional or not will suck the life out of you and resent you for dying. Dare programs around the world taught us in elementary school to, "Just say NO!"

When most people think about love, it's usually an emotion displayed externally toward someone or something. Very seldom, do we as human beings think of love internally, and if we do it's always after we've expressed "love" for other people or things. We live in a society that demand our love while refusing to offer any or acknowledge that women too need love in order to give it. We live in a land that socializes women, especially women of color. The patriarchy of this land disturbs the peace, wreak havoc and incite chaos on the minds, body, and spirit of these women. Women in western civilization live among people that fosters insecurity, invalidates feelings, minimize experiences and marginalize women. Women are taught very early to hate ourselves first and then each other. For women carrying several crosses of intersectionality, their very existence is threatened. I agree with Lisa Vallejos, a blogger for Elephantjournal.com in that, "The battle wages on and as we all know, we are needed to survive. We have important work to do and we need to be okay ourselves to be able to support others. There is no shame in acknowledging you need a break and some support. In fact, it takes great courage to say, "I'm not okay," and to receive the help that is offered. Part of our commitment to doing healing work in the world is found in doing healing work within." Making the decision to love and care for ourselves is revolutionary and necessary. For me, the decision was made at the realization that I wasn't meant to survive.

Self-Preservation is only one element of self-care. It is here that we learn to prioritize what we feel, need and desire ahead of others. Self-preservation carves out time in your daily lives that allow us to pour into yourself what you so freely and selflessly give to the world. Taking the time love on you, ignites healing. Self-love closes the wounds and covers the scrapes acquired just by waking up daily. It protects and covers the heart allowing you to recharge, restore, release and relax. It deepens your understanding of yourself and the world around you. It fine tunes your intuition and decision making. Self-Love petitions a reservoir that allows you to tap into your own power and manifest the highest form of yourself.

The pages to follow will take a closer look at self-care, equitable and accessible self-care practices and deliver check points to ensure that YOU, are taking proper care of yourself and that you are loving yourself in a way that you would want others to love you.

Chapter 2: Ommm My Gawd: First Steps in Self Care

For many of us women, most of our lives have been one big hate fest.... Now hear me out before you begin to scowl your face, smack your lips and roll your eyes. Seriously consider, the notion that we have single-handedly participated if not aid in the creation of this hate fest. How many times have you said, "I'm top fat, or I'm too dark, or light, or skinny or mean"? Women have made it their business to torture and tear down themselves by comparing themselves to other women. It could be the appearance of another woman, the partner that another woman has, the number of children or lack of children, the length of her hair, position of her nose, the spread of her lips, the curve in her hips.... No matter what another woman has or doesn't have we are in constant chaos examining our own lives against that of someone else's. Our self-talk is so brutal. Often times we don't realize that we are doing this, yet we often wonder what's wrong with us...based on the world outside of us. And to be honest, we need to STOP IT!

How can we command someone else to see our worth when we are our own worst critic? A very interesting thing happens when we think and speak so negatively of ourselves. Others begin to mirror and dispense the energy that they receive from you. That's right we are so powerful that we project our feelings and thoughts onto others. If you've ever been uncomfortable with your appearance, felt that your accomplishments were shallow or undeserved, felt that the break up or divorce was solely your fault or even worse self-sabotaged things in your life then its no doubt that you too have fallen for far down negativity's dark hole.

This my friends puts you in a position to care for yourself that much more! You can't expect someone to see the beauty in you, if you don't see the beauty in you. Your self-worth is reflected in the things you speak and do, the people you associate yourself with, the places and circumstances you allow yourself to be in, and the reaction to those things that you simply can't control. It's imperative that you speak to yourself in the way that you would speak to your children or would want someone else to speak to you. Not only is it imperative it is empowering and powerful to recognize that self-hate is brutal, hinders your productivity, but that it also takes you into a deeper much harder to crawl out of sunken place. Now is the time to retrain that thought process. There are several steps one must consistently take to start on the fast track to proper self-care. In this chapter, I will discuss a few steps to help get you started. It is important for you to understand that this isn't a get healed quick challenged. Self-care is an ongoing process that must be done for the rest of your life to ensure that you live your best life.

Step 1: Watch Your Mouth and Your Thoughts- Be Impeccable with them.

I happen to be an avid reader of Don Miguel Ruiz. I have under my belt several of his books that have urged me along in my self-care journey. The most profound book of his that I have read is the Four Agreements. Of the agreements discussed, the most insightful is, be impeccable with your words. Seems simple right? Perhaps on the surface, it is, but as you begin to practice this daily you become more cognizant of the things you speak to yourself and others, the place from which you speak them, and the healing that will come from them. This is where things have a tendency to get complicated. Gary Van Warmerdam, a teacher of Toltec Wisdom states,

"The expression of your Word is much more than just the expression of your words. Your word (small case) has to do with the things you say. They make up sentences, phrases that you speak and write. They come out as opinions, or comments, thoughts in your head, or could even make it into policy in some situations. On the other hand your Word is much more. Your Word (upper case) has to do with the power you have to create through every kind of expression you make. You create through multiple types of expression including emotions, attitude, actions, what you refrain from, and what you express your faith in.

You can create how you feel emotionally by generating emotions, and then you feel them. You can create dynamics of respect in relationship by being silent and listening attentively. You can create a different experience for yourself and others by refraining from an emotional reaction. You create an income for yourself by how well you express caring in the activity of your work. You create a different self-image of yourself by putting the power of your faith in a thought you have about yourself. This can happen in a very subtle and almost passive way of just accepting what you think about yourself as true. You express in a multitude of ways throughout the day and being impeccable with your Word applies to all of them."

Your words create your world. Your thoughts become things. What you say creates your story. Think about it for a moment....don't worry, I'll wait, I have time for it today. This reminds me of the oracle scene from the matrix when she warns him against breaking the vase, and then after he breaks it says to the tune of," I wonder if I had not said anything, would you have broken it." What's important to remember here is, that what we say can and will manifest the more we believe it. The force of life is in all of the things we do, say and feel. The goal is to share with you how to create a story that is drafted with truth and love. Truth is, you are worth it. You deserve your best life and to be surrounded with people that operate in love. Truth is, there is no better person than to create that with than you!

Step 2: Declutter EVERYTHING!

Now that you are well on your way to proper self-care and creating a life that no one deserves more than you with impeccable words/Words you may find yourself running across things and people that should have never been allowed in your space. That's perfectly ok, the universe grants us all permission to rid ourselves of common and proper nouns that no longer serve us. Decluttering is a very necessary part of self-care and is the one practical thing you can do to help improve your life.

If you're as sentimental as I am, then you keep everything from that poem you wrote to your ex-boyfriend during your freshman year of high school to the six pregnancy tests that confirmed growth of your first born who happens to be 18 years old now. Sure those things meant something, but the time had arrived to detach and let go. Just like we are often unaware of the effects of our words, we often ignore or discount the energy that we attach to things. Clutter drains your energy and has a negative effect on your physical, mental and emotional banks. For example, how many times have you heard a song, which totally kills the good mood you have been dying to be in for days because it nudges a memory that depletes our energy levels? It's time to face those things and then let them go. Clutter stagnates your energy and energy flow. Dust is a perfect indicator

People have the tendency to push to the back of their minds and hearts those things that have hurt us or caused us pain and discomfort. Those same people have a tendency to revisit similar situations and attract the likeness of old people in new people and wonder why. The answer is, YOU!. The universe is a pretty good instructor and will give you the same lessons over and over again until you pass the test. The cheat code to passing the test is to declutter. Cleaning out contact lists, closets, bags and boxes is a sure fire way to start decluttering. Throwing away those things that remind you of someone you haven't spoken to in years brings a certain level of relief. It doesn't matter if the memory associated to things was good or bad. What you should remember here is that you can't fill your life with new memories if old ones are taking up space. Instead of focusing on the fact that you no longer have that old dress your favorite football player's mother bough you, re-shift your focus on that new dress that you've been wanting and doing things to ensure that you get it.

The things that clutter your thoughts are untruths that we have somehow begun to believe. This includes those thoughts and words that we speak and absorb. These things often induce fear, regret and any other notion that prevents us from properly caring for ourselves. This clutter has us feeling distracted and unable to relax...both key factors in self-care. Clutter bombards our minds with excessive stimuli that cause our minds to work overtime. This leads to stress that can begin to manifest itself physically. The dust around things is symbolic of stagnant energy. This inhibits our ability to move forward. If at work you are lazy in your thinking, content, not giving things much thought then how can you acquire the knowledge necessary to elevate your position or increase your salary? Do you not believe you're worthy of a promotion? Are you afraid of excelling and being appreciated for your dedication and a job well done? Declutter those thoughts and things that keep you in the same position that you've been in for the last two or more years. I'd like to think that growth is consistent and at the end of two years you should naturally be ready for more, however if its longer then decluttering is essential.

Step 3: Affirming Yourself

According to dictionary definition, to "affirm" something means that you are declaring it as truth. It is those things that we speak as if they are already happening. As we speak those things we begin to carry out tasks to make those things true. For instance, if you say that you are by your definition of "fine" then you will begin to do things to ensure that happens like monitor what you eat, take more steps in a day, plan to work out and seek out information that fits your ability and willingness. An affirmation is a statement that is on repeat to make an assertion to yourself and more of a declaration to the universe that your intention will manifest. According to Eve Hogan, a Spirituality and Health blogger this occurs because of Reticular Activating System (RAS), which is a filter that allows in information that we need and flushes out information that we don't need by using the repetition of those things that we speak and think as important. Using affirming language and statements sends messages to our RAS of what's important. This component of our magnificent brain workings, motivate and lead us to actions to help achieve our goals.

Affirmations makes us uncomfortable in that it creates a conviction within when we are behaving in ways that aren't conducive to higher vibes and positive thoughts. Remember, affirmations are statements of truth and if you are speaking and believing that you are light worker but find yourself cast among gossip, negative talk and energies then that conflicts with your newly designated truths and an opportunity for decluttering exists. Begin by ridding yourself of things, people and spaces and then focusing on those things that you wish to achieve using positive language. Negative language usually includes 'no', 'not', and 'can't' statements. Take care to avoid those words in conversation and thought.

Some say that to successfully form a habit takes 21 days. Adopt this notion when you begin affirming yourself. Take it a step further and go 30 full days. Initially, you will have to set reminders for yourself. Some of my favorite are using sticky notes around my room and bathroom. Others include a dry erase or chalk board in high traffic areas such as the kitchen, or by the front door. If you repeat your affirmations daily they will replace the negative things that once consumed your thoughts subconsciously. You will begin to carry out actions, release the things causing you stress, and ensure that your thoughts and actions align. Make your own list of affirmations at the end of this chapter.

Here are few affirming statements and starters that I use:

I am . (beautiful, authentic, peace)

I have

I am have gratitude for/towards

I attract , because I am deserving and worthy.

I speak and act from a place of love everyday, all day.

I forgive (myself)

I see the best in .

This is my .

Positive vibes and good energy are the driving forces in my life.

I create the life I want to live.

My heart is full of love.

Abundance, prosperity and success guides my steps.

Step 4: Manifestation Ideas

At the beginning of every New Year, the world lights up with vision board party invites and self-improvement classes. Everyone is making proclamation on how they will improve their lives in the New Year, as compared to the last. It's all so full of intent. Since it's the beginning of a new you...as you've begin to choose our words more carefully, you've released some things, and begin to affirm yourself so that you feel better and in charge of your own fate, it's important to have a little vision board party of sorts for yourself or with any friends that have begun this journey with you. A critical part of self-care is seeing those things you've only thought about come to fruition knowing that you had every hand in it occurring.

Vision boards help you see those things you've only thought of. I personally, enjoy incorporating a manifestation path or wheel in my vision boards. It usually has a starting point of those things that I deem most important and then a general but natural path for achieving those things. Vision boards and the like confirms the intent set in affirming yourself and sets in motion the law of attraction. Seeing your visions daily keeps them at the forefront of your thoughts and you simultaneously begin seeking information to help those visions come to life. Manifestation boxes is another craft that can be used to attract those things you desire. An old show box or jewelry box can be ladled in newspaper and magazine clippings that commemorate what you are wanting to achieve. You can add to it and get as creative as possible with it. The goal is to fill it with things that you realistically can commit to and obtain. In speaking impeccable words you have already learned that anything is possible simply because you desire it like the air you breathe.

As we are creating our boards and boxes it's all fun. We often get caught up in the idea of the magic of manifestation as if it's simply some wishing well that we can throw a penny in, go to sleep and wake up and all of our dreams have come true. But that's not how it works. I think this portion of manifestation talk is just as important as creating the boards or boxes themselves. As we request things from the universe we often focus on the end result and final outcome...getting what we asked for. We give little thought to the work and sometimes anguish that accompanies greatness. Manifestation work pulls on all aspects of the law of attraction. On your way to achieving you goal you will likely face obstacles. In the work of self-care its critical to NOT take these things personally or as signs that you shouldn't do or won't get it. The obstacles that you face are only part of the whole. Keep in mind that YOU create your circumstances, and may require you to release (declutter) those negative thoughts, as the universe receives your vibrations, spoken or otherwise. Sure some things are beyond our control, but how we respond to them isn't. Take time to reflect, repeat your affirmations, release the bull, refresh your outlook and path and realign yourself with your goal. We find that resisting those things that are uncomfortable and sometimes inevitable causes us the most tension during our self-care journey. It is imperative that we just go with the flow, reminding ourselves along the way that we deserve this, we are important and will do exactly what we say we will.

Self-care is not one set thing, rather it's a plethora of actions, words and thoughts that lead us to creating a better us and life for ourselves and all those whose lives we touch. Explore a variety of ideas and tips and utilize those that work for you. Create your own self-care cocktail if you will. The idea is to get started and never stop. Women have the hard job of creating the world and then saving it from the very people we've birthed into it, oft times that person is one self and if in those few instances that it's not, we must be in a position of healing, love, and truth in order to assist others. Once you've created any resemblance of harmony and peace in your own life, do everything in your power to maintain it by starting with you first.

Chapter 3: Unplug and Play

The words that will follow this sentence may make me some enemies for life and well in this case that's perfectly OK, because it need to be said. Put your phone down, whatever it is can wait! During the initial period of self-care, I highly recommend that you take a social media break for a minimum of 30 days. Social media provides us with connections and more immediate access to information and news. This means we experience the tragedies and trauma of the world as it occurs. Though those things may not affect us directly we are directly impacted as members of the affected community. We unknowingly absorb that energy and feel a range of emotions that if experienced enough can produce symptoms of PTSD and depression. According to Cornell University's Steven Strogatz, social media sites can make it more difficult for us to distinguish between the meaningful relationships we foster in the real world, and the numerous casual relationships formed through social media. By focusing so much of our time and psychic energy on these less meaningful relationships, our most important connections, he fears, will weaken.

Social media colors and skews the creation of the self and how this construction affects our well-being. The ideal self is the self we aspire to be. Continuous exposure to traumatic and seemingly insensitive events and activity on your time line can worsen your life and circumstances. People often report feeling less confident when comparing their lives to that of their social media friends. May I remind us all that people will present idealized versions of themselves and send you searching feverishly for ways to present yours in upward comparison leading to negative emotions. Checking your social media sites in the morning or before bed leads to increased anxiety and discomfort in sleeping patterns and relaxation. Another stark outcome of social media is cyber bullying. Sadly, this is a real phenomenon among adult women of all races. The devastation of these online attacks can leave deep mental scars. In several well-publicized cases, victims have even been driven to suicide. The anonymity afforded online can bring out dark impulses that might otherwise be suppressed. People that we have confided in will tell our darkest secrets if and when "mad day" comes. The last thing women need is another woman 'coming for them' on social media when we are doing our best just like them to hold it all together. Women and people of color are often put in the position to defend their existence and experiences, and while you can't change how people are or what they do, you can eliminate them from your life and the first place to start is disconnecting from social media (Decluttter).

If social media is critical to your work or business then may I suggest creating a schedule for online promotions and advertising, and adhering to that schedule. You will find more time to tend to yourself. Many of us have seen or have been one of those women in public space that burns out over and over because they feel obligated to give everyone their time, and are attacked when they don't. A woman serving herself and her own needs is a radical act in our society, and it overrules others compulsion to express their problems as yours.

Now that you have unplugged, you may be asking what to do next, and I for one am glad that you asked. The answer is simple...get out there and play! Self-care begins with ascertaining where we are mentally and doing what is necessary to create balance and healthy mindsets. It also requires us to take preventative measures when it comes to the care of our bodies. Caring for ourselves generates more energy. One surefire way to increase energy is to attend to our physical selves and incorporate exercise. Now, I know what you're thinking..." I have so many more important things to do on my agenda than exercising." And while I am sure that's true, one of the first things that should be added to your agenda by now is self-care. Basically, the excuses stop here! There are a plethora of ways to get in the exercise and they are accompanied by a myriad of mental and physical benefits.

When you think of exercise, don't think of traditional gym work, although if the gym is your thing then please go. Exercise can come at any time in your day and in many shapes and forms. Waking up 15 minutes earlier than normal is one way to gift yourself time to exercise. After praying, meditating or coffee, do an aerobic activity or cardio for 10-15 minutes. This is will give you a little extra pep in your step and actually motivate you to get in a few extra minutes after you get home for the evening. If you are absolutely not a morning person then I suggest you do that same aerobic or cardio activity after dinner. If exercising in that manner is something that you have to "grow" into here are a few other ways to get in those steps.

Park as far from the employee entrance at your job as possible and comfortable and take those extra steps and time to affirm yourself and your day. If things get tense while you're at work, take a lunch break stroll. It will give you a chance to sort out your feelings and give you a list of ideas toward resolution or peace restoration. Make an effort to do this at least three to five times each week. If you have to drop the kids off at practice of any kind, stick around and use that time to walk around the facility. Consider joining the YMCA or any drop in class near the drop off point that coincides with practice times and make the most of your time and gas. Of course there are more simple things to do daily, take the stairs at work, walk down every aisle at the grocery store, wash your car, garden, mow the lawn, play with the kids, start a neighborhood walk or hop on your treadmill at home. Everyone can take on exercise, especially the adventure seekers and risk takers. Pull out those old pair of skates or bicycle and get moving. Exercise can and should be a pleasurable activity. If you enjoy swimming take daily dips in the neighborhood pool. Join a yoga or martial arts class. There is absolutely nothing wrong with allowing the energy that doesn't belong to travel down your arm through your hand to be released in a punching bag or the air face of someone that could use a wake up kick. The point here is to increase your physical activity as it leads to clarity in your thoughts and strength in your body.

Ok, ok, my goal here isn't to force feed you anything. The goal of exercise is to release those thoughts and things that inhibit and prevent you from living your best life and to equip you with the energy you need to manifest a shift in yourself. There is no authority that knows more about what you need than you! If exercise is totally NOT your thing then may I suggest that you make a statement! Create something that expresses how you feel. Get out of your head and get busy. The arts are a great way to release things that are subconsciously blocking us. Crafts, writing, poetry, drawing and the like can be productive ways to spend your time and act as tools to healing and caring. Art can have similar effects on your mental and physical effects on your body as exercising. Quilting can be and easy and efficient way to change your focus as it's a way to celebrate life and those happy times in our lives. Drawing can act as a graphic novel of your experiences and as the author you can draft the ending your desire and deserve. Writing can act as a pool where all those things that make us toxic can be released and flushed once you've finished. It, along with poetry can also be a tool in affirming and manifesting those things in your life that will lead you to your best life.

When preparing to unplug and play, I used guiding questions that helped me plan my 'stayscape.' Here are a few questions to assess where and how you need to start: (Be honest in your responses)

1. Do you focus more on what others are doing rather than what you are or could be doing? Why?

2. Do you struggle to find time for exercise? Sleep? Outdoor time? How often do you stretch?

3. When was the last time you got a massage? What's the date and time of your next/first massage?

4. What kind of movement makes you happy? How regularly do you do it? When do you plan to do it again?

5. Do you feel in touch with your sexuality? What things will you do to get in touch with your sexuality?

6. How much time do you spend sitting in front of a computer or with your phone in your hand every day?

7. When was the last time you were alone for an extended period of time without being productive (cooking, cleaning, running errands etc.)? How did that make you feel?

8. How often do you sit in silence without technology (phone, TV, computer)?

9. How often do you feel overwhelmed?

10. When do you feel most at peace? How can you be there, doing that more of the time?

11. Do you enjoy being in your own company? Why?/Why Not?

Chapter 4: The Year of Me: Restoration

So by now, you should have gone through a range of emotions. Self-Care forces us to deal with those things about ourselves that we don't like and to fix them. If you're caring for yourself following this guide, or not, you have compiled a list; written or mental of things that you know you must let go. Once we let go of things we often don't know that we have to fill those holes. Here is where intent and manifestation meet. This is where you restore thoughts and actions with more desirable ones. Once you've carved out time just for you… may I suggest that you give yourself one continuous year of self-care. This doesn't mean you have to follow a traditional year (January to December). Your year can start from the date you started reading this book. This chapter has been organized in seasons, though the work can be done at any time you see fit. Make this year the year that you learn to say NO to anything that makes you roll your eyes, smack your teeth or disturb your peace. Remember, self-care is a non-negotiable.

"We cannot stop the winter or the summer from coming. We cannot stop the spring or the fall or make them other than they are. They are gifts from the universe that we cannot refuse. But we can choose what we will contribute to life when each arrives."- Gary Zukav

There are seasons in our lives that we move at the speed of light. For women that's most of the seasons in our lives. The key to surviving these seasons and maintain our levels of care requires rejuvenation and restoration.

Winter-"The pine stays green in winter...wisdom in hardship." –Norman Doulgas

Ahh the biting cold, warm soup and a seemingly large amount of down time. The winter is a time that we reflect. Here is where you let go those things that you have been holding on to that haven't bothered to hold on to you, to serve you in the way that you deserve. In the winter I find it easier to examine the previous seasons and determine what worked well and what didn't. I use that reflection to release, renew and plan for the upcoming seasons. Winter is a good time to revisit and realign your affirmations to the growth that you have thus far and the growth that you will achieve in the future. Make a few of those affirmations your mantra for this season. It will help you refocus your purpose in this season.

Spring- "No matter how long winter is, spring is sure to follow"- Proverb

The spring is a symbol of rebirth and renewal. Winter has just passed and you have let some things go and found more serving and positive things to fill those voids that you've held on to. Here is where we start generating energy. Clearing old spaces, reorganizing your home and thoughts are done in this season. And while, decluttering is a continuous process, take care during this season get to those things that you've been putting off. Use the spring energy to learn and progress. Revisit and complete those tasks that you were in the middle of but got pulled away from. Finish writing that book, or finalize that proposal and present it to your boss. Nurture existing friendships. With all of this self-love you have been giving yourself, they are probably feeling a bit neglected, and because your friends are extensions of you, you want to make sure that you put some of that love back into the people that have been supporting your through your journey. I would even say the spring is a good time to take up new interest. Go out and meet people. Find those that are walking the new path you've taken. Bond with people new and old that you can draw inspiration from. Attend a workshop or travel to a new place in your state. Spontaneity is definitely one of the biggest contributors to happiness and self-knowing. Be open to new opportunities and try to change up your schedule.

Flowers grow in the spring and so will you.

Summer: "Summertime is always the best of what might be. "- Charles Bowden

The summer time is full of sun energy. The days are longer and the sun shine dissolves the shadows in our lives. This is one of the most important seasons in self- care. Its symbolic of vitality. This is a time where it is all about YOU and saying "No" is a perfectly complete sentence. Saying no to things that you just don't want to do, invest the energy in will free up the time and space for you to do exactly what you want to do. Consider what happens when you say "NO" to things that don't vibe with you, excite you, or work with your schedule. Saying "NO" is the ultimate form of self-care. The summertime is a perfect time to introduce your change(s) to the people around you. Let them know what your boundaries are and if you care to offer an explanation then do so. Here is also a time to seek out resources for those areas that need improvement. Take your self-care to the next level. Start meditating or growing deeper in your mediation. Join meditation circles. Its important to understand that though you are doing things by yourself, for yourself, you are not alone. Connecting with other people to expand your growth is just as important to your self-care path as spending time alone and self-preservation.

Fall: "Life starts all over again when it gets crisp in the fall"- F. Scott Fitzgerald

The fall is absolutely one of my favorite seasons of the year simply because of the crisp air. Autumn is the season of transition and culmination. During this time, this is where significant progress can be seen on your self-care path. There is pride and honor in your journey. All of the affirming and manifestation that you have done is coming to be so in your life. Now that you have said "No" because it's a complete sentence, the fall is a perfect time to incorporate "yes" into your dialogue. It is time to challenge yourself in ways that you haven't been able to because you didn't know how. I'm not talking about filling up all that space that you've worked so diligently to clean out. This isn't a request to become a 'yes' woman, rather it's a nudge to say yes to those things that you were afraid of, didn't have the confidence to face, and yes to doing those things that will take you to the next level of your life.

Restoration is defined as the act of reinstating/bringing back to a former position or condition. The main goal in the restoration process will be to uproot any negative or destructive issues that are causing you unhappiness and pain. With self-restoration comes limitless opportunities. Once you have confidence in your surroundings and yourself, you'll find happiness, break down the walls built by stereotypes and, most importantly, promote your authentic self.

CHAPTER 5: FINALLY, BACK TO ME!

Let's face it, there are barriers to caring for ourselves, and overcoming those barriers are pretty difficult, especially for women. Yet, it's imperative for us to make time and create space for ourselves. It's essential to our existence and well-being and for those that share space with us daily. It easy for us to lose the notion of self-care amid the age of cell-phones, entitled people, dependent children, impatient bosses and demanding spouses. Our natural response is to place our needs at the bottom of tasks that need attention. Self-care is a task that we must tend to just as proper rest and employment. There is absolutely nothing more important than caring for yourself. We need to address the idea that self-sacrifice is natural to those of us that are caregivers, wives and the like. Because of the nurturing parts of ourselves we tend to feel guilt and attach the label of being selfish. However, foregoing our own needs can put an added strain on relationships with those you love. It can lead to resentment, bitterness, and exhaustion. I, personally insist, on being selfish. It's your right, when you live most days of your life being selfless.

Disregarding our own needs while meeting the needs of those around us can gravely impact our mental, physical, spiritual and emotional health. Stress heightens risks for heart problems and even cancer. Not eating healthy or exercising regularly increases chances of suffering from chronic health problems. In addition, lack of self-care can lead to anxiety, depression and render us less productive.

There are also sociological effects with being a "strong woman" more importantly, a "strong black woman". As mothers we are raising girls that are watching us and mimicking our every move. This puts us in a place to see the effects of not caring for ourselves. Do you want to leave that legacy for your daughter? I have to wonder why we do this. We don't receive anything for being selfless. There is no award or extension on our lives. Only resentment. This is a dangerous legacy to leave behind. It perpetuates the vicious cycle of putting others needs above our own. It is up to us to teach them better.

There are also profound spiritual losses when we submerge our own needs and desires and let everyone else's expectations float to the surface. Anna Quindlen describes it well in her book, *Being Perfect* (Random House, 2005), "Someday, sometime, you will be sitting somewhere...And something bad will have happened: You will have lost someone you loved, or failed at something at which you badly wanted to succeed. And sitting there, you will fall into the center of yourself. You will look for some core to sustain you. And if you have been perfect all your life and have managed to meet all of the expectations of your family, your friends, your community, your society, chances are that there will be a black hole where that core ought to be. (Martin, C. 2008)

Self-care is about getting to the core of yourself, centering and strengthening properly. It's about listening to your body's demands and understanding that you can't care for anyone else correctly without properly caring for yourself. Remember, please place the oxygen mask on yourself before assisting other passengers. Now go on, reclaim your time and care for yourself like you do for everyone else.

CITATIONS

This book was written in part with insight and/or direct quotes from the following sources:

Side Note This list of citations doesnt follow any governing body of literary rules.

http://www.dsausa.org/black_bodies_self_care_and_the_limits_of_cla

http://www.thefeministwirc.com/2014/04/self-love-and-self-care/

http://spiritualityhealth.com/blog/eve-hogan/affirmations-why-they-work-how-use-them

http://reneelongworth.com/day-2-of-365-days-of-feng-shui-decluttering/

https://experiencelife.com/article/the-art-of-self-care/

http://www.somatics.de/artikel/for-professionals/2-article/43-the-tao-of-exercise-and-self-care

http://www.toltecspirit.com/four-agreements/impeccable-word/

http://www.thefeministwire.com/2012/11/subversive-self-care-centering-black-womens-wellness/

https://www.psychologytoday.com/blog/the-fallible-mind/201204/no-is-complete-sentence

MEET THE AUTHOR

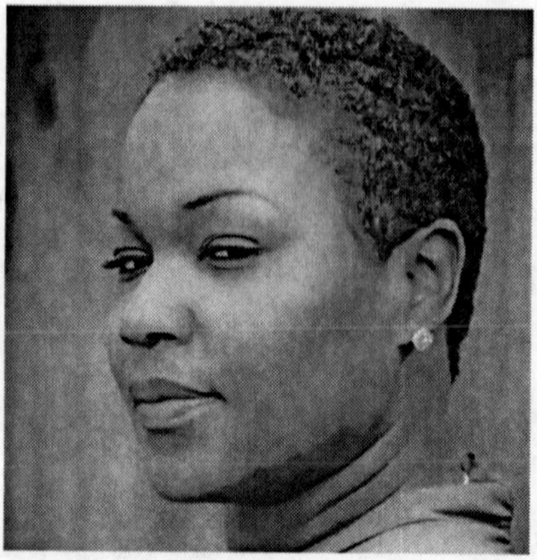

Jeanette MsNightLyfe Ferrell is a breath of fresh air. Ms. Nightlyfe is a published columnist, author, motivational speaker and international poet. Her poetic accolades includes international work with SpokenWord Paris [http://spokenwordparis.org/] in Paris, France and Vortex [http://www.sofraiche.com/floacists-poetry-night/] in London with Natalie Stewart (Floacist) of Floetry. She is a former associate producer and member of The Punany Poets, from HBO's Real Sex. As the founder of Sweet Tooth Media, and Editor-In-Chief of the The S.W.E.E.T Magazine, she has created positive press for several trendsetters and culture shocking revolutionaries such as San Francisco and Atlanta Black Prides, Nishia Da Diva Productions, Amuse Bourche Entertainment, K. Dapree's he(ART) and Soul, Entertainer Butterfly Soul, Pride Books and more. She has an MBA from LeTourneau University, Bachelor of Science from Texas Wesleyan University and is pursuing a MA in School Psychology from Howard University. She currently resides in Washington, D.C. with her wife and youngest of two sons.

Follow her on
FB/Twitter: @MsNightLyfe
IG: @NightLyfes_Venom
Web: www.SweetToothMedia.com [http://www.SweetToothMedia.com]

CPSIA information can be obtained
at www.ICGtesting.com
Printed in the USA
FFOW02n1519200118
44599799-44487FF

9 781499 903430